STROKE DIET RECIPES FOOD LIST

Wholesome Healing: Nourishing Recipes for Stroke Recovery and Lifelong Wellness

Daniel J. Contreras

Table of Contents

Introduction:

The Power of Food After a Stroke

A stroke is a life-changing event, and the path to recovery requires a multi-faceted approach. While medical care plays a crucial role, what you put on your plate can have a profound impact on your healing journey. Food serves as the fuel for your body's remarkable ability to repair and regenerate. By making smart dietary choices, you can actively participate in your recovery, promoting:

- **Tissue Repair:** The right nutrients provide the building blocks for your body to rebuild damaged tissues in your brain and throughout your body.
- **Improved Blood Flow:** Consuming heart-healthy foods can help regulate blood pressure and cholesterol, reducing the risk of future strokes.

- **Enhanced Brain Function:** Specific nutrients can support cognitive function and memory, aiding in regaining lost abilities.

- **Overall Well-being**: A balanced diet rich in vitamins, minerals, and antioxidants strengthens your immune system and promotes overall health.

Building a Foundation for Lifelong Wellness

While the immediate focus after a stroke is naturally on recovery, this is also an opportunity to establish healthy habits that will benefit you for years to come. The dietary principles that promote healing after a stroke are, in many ways, the same principles that support long-term well-being. By embracing a stroke diet, you're laying the groundwork for a healthy lifestyle that can:

- **Reduce Your Risk of Recurrence:** Maintaining a balanced diet with limited sodium, saturated fat, and added sugars can significantly lower the risk of another stroke.

- **Promote Heart Health:** Eating a heart-healthy diet keeps your arteries clear and supports healthy blood pressure, reducing strain on your cardiovascular system.

- **Maintain Cognitive Function:** Certain nutrients play a vital role in brain health. By incorporating these foods regularly, you can help prevent cognitive decline and support memory function.

- **Boost Energy Levels:** The right balance of carbohydrates, protein, and healthy fats provides sustained energy throughout the day, helping you stay active and engaged in life.

- **Improve Overall Quality of Life:** A healthy diet contributes to better sleep, improved mood, and a stronger immune system, all of which significantly impact your overall well-being.

This section emphasizes the long-term benefits of a stroke diet. It highlights how these dietary changes not only support recovery but also contribute to a healthier and more fulfilling life.

Part 1: Essential Stroke Recovery Foods

The first phase of your stroke recovery journey requires providing your body with the essential nutrients it needs to heal and rebuild. This section delves into the five key food groups that form the foundation of a stroke recovery diet:

- **Fruits and Vegetables:** Nature's powerhouses of vitamins, minerals, and antioxidants, fruits and vegetables play a vital role in recovery.

They provide essential vitamins for nerve function, fiber for gut health, and antioxidants to combat inflammation.

- **Whole Grains:** Whole grains offer a slow and steady release of energy, crucial for supporting your body's healing processes. They are also rich in fiber, which helps regulate blood pressure and cholesterol.

- **Lean Protein:** Protein is the building block for tissue repair. Lean protein sources like fish, poultry, and legumes provide the essential amino acids your body needs to rebuild damaged tissues and support muscle function.

- **Low-Fat Dairy:** Low-fat dairy products are a valuable source of calcium and vitamin D, both of which are essential for bone health and recovery. They offer protein and other necessary nutrients as well.

- **Healthy Fats:** Don't be afraid of fat! Healthy fats like those found in avocados, olive oil, nuts, and seeds play a crucial role in brain health and function. They also promote satiety and help with nutrient absorption.

Each chapter within this section will explore these food groups in detail, highlighting their specific benefits for stroke recovery. You'll also find sample recipes that are not only delicious but also easy to prepare and follow, considering any swallowing or chewing difficulties you might be experiencing.

Chapter 1: Fruits and Vegetables: Nature's Powerhouse of Nutrients

Fruits and vegetables are the cornerstones of a healthy stroke recovery diet. They are packed with essential vitamins, minerals, and antioxidants that play a vital role in healing and overall well-being.

Benefits of Fruits and Vegetables for Stroke Recovery:

- **Rich in Vitamins and Minerals:** Fruits and vegetables provide a wide range of vitamins and minerals, including vitamins A, C, E, and K, as well as potassium and magnesium. These nutrients are essential for nerve function, muscle health, and immune system support, all of which are crucial for stroke recovery.

- **Antioxidant Powerhouse:** Fruits and vegetables are brimming with antioxidants that help combat free radicals in the body. Free radicals can damage cells and contribute to inflammation, which can hinder healing after a stroke.

- **Fiber for Gut Health:** Stroke recovery can sometimes lead to digestive issues. The fiber found in fruits and vegetables promotes gut health and regularity, aiding in a smoother recovery process.

- **Hydration:** A lot of fruits and vegetables are high in water, which aids in maintaining your fluid balance.Proper hydration is essential for overall health and can improve blood flow, which is important for stroke recovery.

Incorporating Fruits and Vegetables into Your Stroke Diet:

- **Variety is Key:** Aim for a rainbow on your plate! Include fruits and vegetables of different colors to ensure you're getting a wide range of nutrients.

- **Fresh, Frozen, or Canned (Low Sodium):** All forms of fruits and vegetables can be part of your stroke diet. Fresh options offer the most nutrients, but frozen and canned (low-sodium) varieties are convenient and still provide valuable vitamins and minerals.

- **Think Beyond Salads:** While salads are a great option, explore different ways to incorporate fruits and vegetables into your meals.

- Try smoothies, roasted vegetables, fruit salsas, or adding them to soups and stews.

Recipes:

- **Morning Power Smoothie:** This smoothie is packed with antioxidants and essential vitamins to jumpstart your day.

- **Rainbow Veggie Roast:** Roasting vegetables is a simple and delicious way to bring out their natural sweetness. This recipe is a colorful and flavorful side dish.

- **Fruity Salsa with Baked Chicken:** This salsa adds a burst of freshness to lean protein, making it a satisfying and nutritious meal.

Smoothies, Salads, Roasted Vegetables

Morning Power Smoothie:

This smoothie is a powerhouse of nutrients, perfect for a quick and delicious breakfast or snack.

Ingredients:

- 1 cup frozen berries (blueberries, raspberries, strawberries)
- ½ banana, frozen
- ½ cup plain low-fat yogurt
- ½ cup low-fat milk (or plant-based milk)
- Handful of baby spinach
- ¼ teaspoon ground cinnamon

Instructions:

1. Blend all ingredients together in a blender until they are creamy and smooth.
2. Add a splash of water or milk if needed to achieve desired consistency.
3. Serve immediately and enjoy!

Rainbow Veggie Roast:

Roasting is a simple way to prepare delicious and nutritious vegetables. This recipe allows you to customize it with your favorite veggies.

Ingredients:

- 1 head broccoli, cut into florets
- 1 red bell pepper, sliced
- 1 yellow bell pepper, sliced
- 1 medium zucchini, sliced
- 1 red onion, cut into wedges
- 2 tablespoons olive oil
- ½ teaspoon dried oregano
- Salt and pepper to taste

Instructions:

1. Preheat the oven to 400°F (200°C).

2. In a large bowl, toss vegetables with olive oil, oregano, salt, and pepper.

3. Spread vegetables on a baking sheet in a single layer.

4. Roast for 20-25 minutes, or until vegetables are tender-crisp and slightly browned.

5. Serve hot and enjoy!

Fruity Salsa with Baked Chicken:

This refreshing salsa adds a burst of flavor to lean protein, making it a vibrant and healthy meal.

Ingredients:

- 1 cup chopped tomatoes
- ½ cup chopped mango
- ¼ cup chopped red onion
- 1 tablespoon chopped fresh cilantro
- 1 tablespoon lime juice
- Salt and pepper to taste

For Baked Chicken:

- 2 boneless, skinless chicken breasts
- 1 tablespoon olive oil
- ½ teaspoon dried thyme
- Salt and pepper to taste

Instructions:

Salsa:

1. In a medium bowl, combine tomatoes, mango, red onion, cilantro, and lime juice.
2. Season with salt and pepper to taste.
3. Set aside.

Baked Chicken:

1. Preheat the oven to 400°F (200°C).
2. In a small bowl, combine olive oil, thyme, salt, and pepper.
3. Rub the mixture onto the chicken breasts.
4. Place chicken on a baking sheet lined with parchment paper.
5. Bake for 20-25 minutes, or until cooked through.
6. Serve chicken with a dollop of fruity salsa and enjoy!

Chapter 2: Whole Grains: Fueling Your Body for Recovery

Whole grains are the unsung heroes of a stroke recovery diet. They provide a sustained source of energy, essential for your body's healing processes. Unlike refined grains that are stripped of their nutrients, whole grains offer a powerhouse of benefits:

- **Slow and Steady Energy Release:** Whole grains are rich in complex carbohydrates, which break down slowly in your body, providing a sustained source of energy throughout the day. This is crucial for supporting your body's repair and recovery efforts.

- **Fiber Powerhouse:** Whole grains are packed with fiber, which keeps you feeling full and satisfied, aids in digestion, and helps regulate blood sugar levels.

- **Essential Nutrients:** Whole grains are a valuable source of B vitamins, which play a vital role in energy metabolism and nervous system function. They also offer important minerals like magnesium and iron, which are essential for overall health.

Including Whole Grains in Your Stroke Diet:

- **Make the Switch:** Replace refined grains like white bread, pasta, and rice with whole-grain alternatives. Opt for brown rice, quinoa, whole-wheat bread and pasta, barley, and oats.

- **Start Your Day Right:** Whole grains are a great way to fuel your mornings. Try oatmeal with berries and nuts, whole-wheat toast with avocado, or a quinoa breakfast bowl with fruit and yogurt.

- **Think Beyond the Obvious:** Whole grains can be incorporated throughout your meals. Add cooked quinoa to salads, use whole-wheat breadcrumbs for casseroles, or enjoy brown rice pilaf as a side dish.

Quinoa Bowls, Brown Rice Pilaf, Whole-Wheat Pancakes

This section will showcase a few delicious and easy-to-digest recipes featuring whole grains:

- **Quinoa Power Bowl:** This customizable bowl allows you to pack in protein, vegetables, and whole grains for a complete and satisfying meal.

- **Brown Rice Pilaf with Herbs:** A flavorful side dish that compliments any protein source.

- **Whole-Wheat Pancakes with Berries:** A healthy twist on a classic breakfast favorite.

Quinoa Bowls, Brown Rice Pilaf, Whole-Wheat Pancakes

Quinoa Power Bowl:

This customizable bowl allows you to create a delicious and nutritious meal packed with protein, vegetables, and whole grains. It's a great option for lunch or dinner and can be easily adapted to your preferences and dietary needs.

Ingredients:

- 1 cup cooked quinoa
- ½ cup roasted vegetables (such as broccoli, Brussels sprouts, or sweet potato)
- 4 ounces grilled chicken breast, chopped (or other lean protein)
- ¼ cup crumbled feta cheese (optional)
- 2 tablespoons chopped fresh herbs (such as parsley or cilantro)

- 1 tablespoon olive oil

- Lemon juice to taste

- Salt and pepper to taste

Instructions:

1. Prepare the quinoa according to package instructions.

2. While the quinoa cooks, roast your chosen vegetables.

3. Grill or cook your preferred lean protein source.

4. In a large bowl, combine cooked quinoa, roasted vegetables, chopped protein, feta cheese (if using), and fresh herbs.

5. Olive oil, lemon juice, salt, and pepper should all be combined in a small basin. Shake to coat the bowl after drizzling it with dressing.

6. Serve immediately and enjoy!

Brown Rice Pilaf with Herbs:

This flavorful pilaf is a versatile side dish that compliments any protein source. The use of broth adds depth of flavor, while the herbs provide a fresh touch.

Ingredients:

- 1 cup brown rice
- 1 ½ cups vegetable broth
- 1 tablespoon olive oil
- ½ onion, chopped
- 1 clove garlic, minced
- ½ teaspoon dried thyme
- ¼ cup chopped fresh parsley
- Salt and pepper to taste

Instructions:

1. Olive oil should be heated over medium heat in a medium saucepan. Add the onion and simmer for about 5 minutes, or until softened.
2. Add the garlic and thyme and simmer for a minute more.
3. Add brown rice and stir to coat with oil and spices.
4. Add the veggie broth and season with the pepper and salt.Bring to a boil, then reduce heat to low, cover, and simmer for 45 minutes, or until rice is cooked through and fluffy.
5. Fluff the rice with a fork and stir in fresh parsley before serving.

Whole-Wheat Pancakes with Berries:

A healthy twist on a classic breakfast favorite! These pancakes are packed with whole-grain goodness and can be enjoyed with your favorite toppings.

Ingredients:

- 1 cup whole-wheat flour
- 1 ½ teaspoons baking powder
- ¼ teaspoon salt
- 1 cup milk (or plant-based milk)
- 1 egg
- 1 tablespoon melted butter (or oil)
- ½ cup fresh or frozen berries

Instructions:

1. Mix the flour, baking powder, and salt in a big bowl.

2. In a separate bowl, combine milk, egg, and melted butter.

3. Add the wet ingredients to the dry ingredients and mix until just combined (a few lumps are okay).

4. Gently fold in the berries.

5. Heat a pan or griddle that has been gently oiled over medium heat.

6. Spoon half a cup of batter onto each pancake griddle.

7. Cook for 2 to 3 minutes on each side, or until well cooked and golden brown.

8. Serve immediately with your favorite toppings like maple syrup, fresh fruit, or yogurt.

Chapter 3: Lean Protein: Building and Repairing Tissues

Lean protein is the cornerstone of a stroke recovery diet. After a stroke, your body needs the essential building blocks – amino acids – found in protein to repair and rebuild damaged tissues in your brain and throughout your body. Including a variety of lean protein sources in your diet offers numerous benefits:

- **Tissue Repair:** Protein provides the raw materials your body needs to rebuild damaged tissues, promoting healing and recovery.

- **Muscle Support:** Protein plays a crucial role in maintaining and strengthening muscle mass, which can be helpful for regaining lost mobility and improving function.

- **Satiety:** Protein helps you feel full and satisfied, which can aid in weight management and reduce cravings for unhealthy snacks.

- **Immune System Function:** Protein is essential for a healthy immune system, which is important for fighting off infection and promoting overall health.

Choosing Lean Protein Sources for Stroke Recovery:

- **Focus on Variety:** Incorporate a variety of lean protein sources throughout the week to ensure you're getting a complete range of amino acids.

- **Fish:** Fatty fish like salmon, tuna, and mackerel are rich in omega-3 fatty acids, which are beneficial for brain health and overall well-being.

- **Poultry:** Skinless chicken breast and turkey breast are excellent sources of lean protein and are easily digestible.

- **Beans and Legumes:** A plant-based protein powerhouse! Beans, lentils, and chickpeas are affordable, versatile, and packed with fiber, making them a great addition to your diet.

- **Low-Fat Dairy:** Low-fat yogurt and Greek yogurt are good options for incorporating protein and calcium into your meals.

Tips for Those with Swallowing Difficulties:

- **Soft and Easy-to-Chew Options:** Opt for softer protein sources like cooked fish, ground chicken or turkey, scrambled eggs, or tofu.

- **Pureed Options:** If chewing is a challenge, consider pureeing cooked chicken or fish with broth or yogurt for a smooth and easy-to-swallow option.

- **Protein Powders:** With your doctor's approval, protein powders can be a helpful way to ensure you're meeting your protein needs. Choose unflavored or mildly flavored powders that can be blended into smoothies or yogurt.

Baked Salmon, Chicken Stir-Fry, Lentil Soup

This section will showcase delicious and easy-to-prepare recipes featuring lean protein sources:

- **Baked Salmon with Lemon and Herbs:** A simple and flavorful way to enjoy the health benefits of fatty fish.
- **Chicken Stir-Fry with Vegetables**: A quick and customizable meal packed with protein and veggies.
- **Lentil Soup with Whole Wheat Bread:** A hearty and healthy soup that provides both protein and fiber.

Baked Salmon, Chicken Stir-Fry, Lentil Soup

Baked Salmon with Lemon and Herbs:

This recipe offers a simple and flavorful way to enjoy the heart-healthy benefits of fatty fish.

Ingredients:

- 1 salmon filet (4-6 ounces)
- 1 tablespoon olive oil
- ½ lemon, sliced
- 2 sprigs fresh thyme
- Salt and pepper to taste

Instructions:

1. Preheat the oven to 400°F (200°C).

2. Place salmon filet in a baking dish. Add a drizzle of olive oil and season with pepper and salt.

3. Top with lemon slices and thyme sprigs.

4. The salmon should flake easily with a fork after baking for 15 to 20 minutes, depending on how done it is.

5. Serve immediately with roasted vegetables, quinoa, or a side salad.

Chicken Stir-Fry with Vegetables:

This quick and customizable stir-fry is a great weeknight meal packed with protein and veggies.

Ingredients:

- 1 pound boneless, skinless chicken breasts, cut into bite-sized pieces
- 1 tablespoon cornstarch
- 2 tablespoons soy sauce (low-sodium)
- 1 tablespoon vegetable oil
- 2 cups assorted vegetables (such as broccoli florets, sliced bell peppers, snow peas)
- 1 cup chopped onion
- 1 clove garlic, minced
- ½ cup chicken broth (low-sodium)
- 1 tablespoon rice vinegar
- Salt and pepper to taste

Instructions:

1. In a bowl, toss chicken pieces with cornstarch and soy sauce.

2. In a big wok or skillet, heat the oil over medium-high heat. Add chicken and cook until golden brown and cooked through, about 5 minutes. Remove from the pan and set aside.

3. Add vegetables and onion to the pan and cook for 3-4 minutes, or until softened and slightly crisp-tender.

4. Add the garlic and simmer for one more minute after stirring..

5. Pour in chicken broth and rice vinegar. Bring to a simmer and cook until slightly thickened, about 2 minutes.

6. Return chicken to the pan and toss to coat with the sauce.

7. Season with salt and pepper to taste.

8. Serve immediately over brown rice or quinoa.

Lentil Soup with Whole Wheat Bread:

This hearty and healthy soup provides both protein and fiber, making it a satisfying and nutritious meal. It can be easily adapted for those with swallowing difficulties.

Ingredients:

- 1 tablespoon olive oil
- 1 onion, chopped
- 2 cloves garlic, minced
- 1 cup brown lentils, rinsed
- 4 cups vegetable broth (low-sodium)

- 1 (14.5 oz) can diced tomatoes, undrained

- 1 teaspoon dried thyme

- ½ teaspoon dried oregano

- Salt and pepper to taste

For Serving:

- Whole-wheat bread, toasted or chopped (optional)

- Fresh parsley, chopped (optional)

Instructions:

1. In a big pot, warm up the olive oil over medium heat. Add the onion and simmer for about 5 minutes, or until softened.

2. Add the garlic and simmer for one more minute after stirring.

3. Add lentils, vegetable broth, diced tomatoes, thyme, and oregano. Bring to a boil, then reduce heat to low, cover, and simmer for 30-35 minutes, or until lentils are tender.

4. Season with salt and pepper to taste.

Serving Options:

- **Regular Consistency:** Serve the soup as is with a slice of whole-wheat bread for dipping.

- **For Difficulty Swallowing:** Puree the soup in a blender or food processor until smooth. Add a splash of water or broth if needed to achieve desired consistency. Top with chopped fresh parsley for garnish.

Chapter 4: Low-Fat Dairy: Essential Nutrients for Strong Bones and Recovery

Low-fat dairy products are valuable allies on your stroke recovery journey. They provide a multitude of essential nutrients that not only contribute to strong bones but also support overall well-being:

- **Rich in Calcium and Vitamin D:** Low-fat dairy products are a top source of calcium, a mineral crucial for building and maintaining strong bones. They are also often fortified with vitamin D, which aids in calcium absorption. Strong bones are essential for overall health and can help prevent future fractures.

- **Protein Powerhouse:** Dairy products like yogurt and Greek yogurt offer a good source of protein, which is necessary for tissue repair and muscle function, both of which are critical for stroke recovery.

- **Other Essential Nutrients**: Low-fat dairy also provides essential vitamins and minerals like potassium, B vitamins, and magnesium, all of which contribute to proper nerve function, healthy blood pressure, and overall well-being.

Incorporating Low-Fat Dairy into Your Stroke Recovery Diet:

- **Variety is Key:** Explore a variety of low-fat dairy options like milk, yogurt, and cheese. Choose plain or low-sugar options whenever possible to limit added sugar intake.

- **Incorporate Throughout the Day:** Enjoy low-fat dairy throughout the day. Start your day with a yogurt parfait, include cheese in a salad for lunch, or have a glass of low-fat milk with dinner.

- **Think Beyond the Obvious:** Low-fat dairy can be incorporated into many dishes. Use low-fat yogurt for dips or smoothies, add grated cheese to soups or casseroles, or enjoy low-fat milk in mashed potatoes.

Tips for Those with Lactose Intolerance:

- **Choose Lactose-Free Options:** Many lactose-free dairy products are now available, offering the same taste and benefits without the lactose.

- **Small Amounts:** If you have mild lactose intolerance, you may be able to tolerate small portions of dairy. Try different things to determine what suits you the best.

- **Calcium Alternatives:** If you cannot tolerate dairy at all, consult your doctor about alternative sources of calcium, such as leafy green vegetables, fortified plant-based milks, and calcium supplements.

Yogurt Parfait, Cottage Cheese with Fruit, Low-Fat Milk in Smoothies

This section will showcase delicious and easy-to-prepare recipes featuring low-fat dairy options:

- **Fruity Yogurt Parfait:** A layered yogurt parfait is a refreshing and nutritious breakfast or snack option.

- **Cottage Cheese with Fruit and Herbs:** A simple and protein-packed snack or light lunch.

- **Berry Smoothie with Low-Fat Milk:** A delicious and healthy smoothie packed with essential nutrients.

Yogurt Parfait, Cottage Cheese with Fruit, Low-Fat Milk in Smoothies

Fruity Yogurt Parfait:

A layered yogurt parfait is a refreshing, customizable, and nutritious breakfast or snack option. It allows you to combine the creaminess of low-fat yogurt with the sweetness and texture of fruit and granola.

Ingredients:

- 1 cup low-fat yogurt (plain or vanilla)
- ½ cup granola
- ½ cup fresh or frozen berries
- ¼ cup chopped nuts (optional)
- Honey or maple syrup to taste (optional)

Instructions:

1. In a small glass or parfait dish, layer half of the yogurt.
2. Top with half of the granola and berries.
3. Repeat layers with remaining yogurt, granola, and berries.
4. Drizzle with honey or maple syrup for additional sweetness (optional).
5. Sprinkle with chopped nuts for added protein and texture (optional).

Cottage Cheese with Fruit and Herbs:

This simple and protein-packed recipe is a great snack or light lunch option. It's easy to prepare and offers a delightful combination of sweet and savory flavors.

Ingredients:

- ½ cup low-fat cottage cheese
- ½ cup chopped fruit (such as mango, pineapple, or peaches)
- 1 tablespoon chopped fresh herbs (such as mint or basil)
- Salt and pepper to taste

Instructions:

1. In a bowl, combine cottage cheese, chopped fruit, and fresh herbs.
2. Add a dash of salt and pepper, according to your taste.
3. Serve immediately and enjoy!

Berry Smoothie with Low-Fat Milk:

This delicious and healthy smoothie is a quick and convenient way to incorporate low-fat dairy and fruit into your diet. It's packed with essential nutrients and can be enjoyed for breakfast, a post-workout snack, or anytime you need a pick-me-up.

Ingredients:

- 1 cup frozen berries (such as blueberries, raspberries, or strawberries)
- ½ cup low-fat milk
- ½ banana, frozen
- ¼ cup plain low-fat yogurt (optional)
- Handful of baby spinach (optional)
- Honey or maple syrup to taste (optional)

Instructions:

1. Combine all ingredients in a blender.
2. Blend until smooth and creamy.
3. Add a splash of water or milk if needed to achieve desired consistency.
4. Serve immediately and enjoy!

Chapter 5: Healthy Fats: Promoting Brain Health and Overall Well-being

While the term "fat" often carries negative connotations, there's a crucial distinction to be made. Healthy fats play a vital role in a stroke recovery diet and overall well-being. In fact, they are essential for promoting brain health and function.

The Power of Healthy Fats for Stroke Recovery:

- **Brain Builders:** Healthy fats, particularly omega-3 fatty acids, are essential building blocks for brain cells. They contribute to cognitive function, memory, and overall brain health.

- **Improved Blood Flow:** Healthy fats may help regulate blood pressure and cholesterol levels, promoting healthy blood flow throughout the body, including the brain.

- **Enhanced Satiety:** Including healthy fats in your diet can help you feel fuller for longer, reducing cravings for unhealthy snacks and supporting weight management.

Choosing the Right Healthy Fats:

- **Unsaturated Fats:** These are the "good" fats and should be a focus of your diet. Examples include monounsaturated fats found in avocados, olive oil, and nuts and polyunsaturated fats found in fatty fish, flaxseeds, and walnuts.

- **Limit Saturated Fats:** Saturated fats, found in red meat, processed meats, and full-fat dairy products, should be limited in a stroke recovery diet.

- **Trans Fats:** Avoid trans fats altogether. These unhealthy fats are often found in fried foods, commercially baked goods, and processed snacks.

Incorporating Healthy Fats into Your Stroke Recovery Diet:

- **Embrace Avocados:** Avocados are a nutritional powerhouse, rich in healthy monounsaturated fats, fiber, and essential vitamins. Enjoy them sliced on toast, mashed into guacamole, or added to salads.

- **Drizzle with Olive Oil:** Olive oil is a versatile and heart-healthy fat. Use it for salad dressings, cooking, or drizzled over roasted vegetables.

- **Snack on Nuts and Seeds:** Nuts and seeds are a convenient source of healthy fats, protein, and fiber. Choose unsalted or dry-roasted varieties for a healthy snack option.

- **Fatty Fish Feast:** Incorporate fatty fish like salmon, tuna, and mackerel into your diet two to three times a week for a rich source of omega-3 fatty acids.

Tips for Those with Difficulty Swallowing:

- **Soft Options:** Choose soft or pureed options like mashed avocado or nut butter.

- **Oil-Based Dressings:** Opt for oil-based salad dressings instead of creamy dressings.

- **Ground Flaxseeds**: Include ground flax
  seeds in smoothies or yogurt for a boost of
  healthy fats.

**Avocado Toast with Eggs, Salmon with
Roasted Vegetables, Trail Mix with Nuts and
Seeds**

This section will showcase delicious and
easy-to-prepare recipes featuring healthy fats:

- **Avocado Toast with Eggs:** A simple and
  satisfying breakfast option packed with
  healthy fats and protein.
- **Baked Salmon with Lemon and Herbs:**
  A classic dish featuring the heart-healthy
  benefits of fatty fish. (You can reference this
  recipe from Chapter 3 for details)

- **Homemade Trail Mix with Nuts and Seeds:** A customizable and portable snack mix brimming with healthy fats, protein, and fiber.

Avocado Toast with Eggs, Salmon with Lemon and Olive Oil, Nut and Seed Trail Mix

Avocado Toast with Eggs:

A simple and satisfying breakfast option packed with healthy fats and protein. This recipe is easily customizable based on your preferences and can be adapted for those with difficulty chewing.

Ingredients:

- 1 slice whole-grain toast
- ½ ripe avocado, mashed
- 2 eggs
- Salt and pepper to taste

- Optional Toppings: Chopped fresh herbs (such as chives or parsley), crumbled feta cheese, hot sauce

Instructions:

1. Toast the whole-grain bread until it reaches the crispness you like.
2. While the bread toasts, cook your eggs according to your preference (fried, scrambled, poached).
3. Over the toast, equally distribute the mashed avocado.
4. Add scrambled eggs on top and season with salt and pepper.
5. Add your favorite toppings for an extra burst of flavor and nutrients.

Swallowing Difficulty Adaptation:

- If chewing is a challenge, consider using a ripe avocado for a smoother mash.
- You can also poach or soft-scramble the eggs for a softer texture.

Salmon with Lemon and Olive Oil:

This recipe showcases the heart-healthy benefits of fatty fish in a simple and flavorful dish. (This recipe builds on the one from Chapter 3 with a focus on healthy fats from olive oil)

Ingredients:

- 1 salmon filet (4-6 ounces)
- 1 tablespoon olive oil
- ½ lemon, sliced
- 2 sprigs fresh thyme
- Salt and pepper to taste

Instructions:

1. Preheat the oven to 400°F (200°C).

2. Place salmon filet in a baking dish.Add a drizzle of olive oil and season with pepper and salt.

3. Top with lemon slices and thyme sprigs.

4. Bake for 15-20 minutes, or until salmon is cooked through and flakes easily with a fork.

5. Serve immediately with roasted vegetables, quinoa, or a side salad.

Nut and Seed Trail Mix:

A customizable and portable snack mix brimming with healthy fats, protein, and fiber. This recipe allows you to control the ingredients and portion sizes.

Ingredients:

- ½ cup unsalted raw almonds
- ¼ cup raw walnuts
- ¼ cup dried cranberries
- ¼ cup pumpkin seeds
- ¼ cup sunflower seeds

Instructions:

1. In a medium bowl, combine all ingredients.

2. Adjust the ingredients and quantities to your preferences. You can include other nuts, seeds, or dried fruits like raisins or chopped dates.

3. Hold for up to a week in an airtight receptacle.

Swallowing Difficulty Adaptation:

- For those with difficulty chewing, opt for pre-chopped nuts and seeds or grind them into a coarser consistency using a mortar and pestle or food processor.

Part 2: Lifelong Wellness Recipes

Building a healthy lifestyle is a journey, and this section equips you with delicious and nutritious recipes that promote overall well-being. These recipes are perfect for everyone, regardless of age or health condition.

We'll explore a variety of dietary principles that contribute to long-term health:

- **Balancing Your Plate**: Mastering the art of creating balanced meals that incorporate all food groups.
- **Plant Power:** Delving into the vast array of plant-based ingredients and their health benefits.

- **Flavorful Cooking with Less Salt:**
  Creating delicious meals without sacrificing
  taste while keeping sodium intake in check.

- **Sweet Treats Done Right:** Indulging in
  healthy and satisfying desserts that won't
  sabotage your wellness goals.

- **Meal Prep Magic:** Planning and preparing
  meals in advance for a stress-free and
  healthy week.

This section provides you with the tools and
inspiration to cook nutritious and flavorful meals
that support lifelong wellness. Get ready to explore
a world of delicious recipes that will tantalize your
taste buds and nourish your body!

Chapter 6: Heart-Healthy Dishes for Continued Recovery

Following a stroke, maintaining a heart-healthy diet is crucial for continued recovery and preventing future complications. This chapter dives into delicious and nutritious recipes that promote cardiovascular health and overall well-being.

These recipes are designed to be:

- **Low in saturated fat:** Limiting saturated fat helps lower bad cholesterol levels, reducing the risk of heart disease.

- **Rich in fiber:** Fiber keeps you feeling full for longer, promotes digestive health, and may help regulate blood sugar levels.

- **Packed with essential nutrients:** These dishes are brimming with vitamins, minerals, and antioxidants that support overall health.

Building Your Heart-Healthy Plate:

The key to a heart-healthy meal is balance. Here's how to create a balanced plate:

- **Half Your Plate:** Fill half your plate with non-starchy vegetables like leafy greens, broccoli, peppers, and mushrooms.
- **One Quarter:** Dedicate a quarter of your plate to lean protein sources like fish, chicken, beans, or lentils.
- **One Quarter:** The remaining quarter can be filled with whole grains such as brown rice, quinoa, or whole-wheat bread.

- **Healthy Fats:** Include a healthy fat source like olive oil, avocado, or nuts for satiety and additional nutrients.

Sample Recipes:

This section offers a variety of delicious and heart-healthy recipes to get you started:

- Mediterranean Chicken with Roasted Vegetables: A classic combination of lean protein, colorful vegetables, and heart-healthy olive oil.
- Lentil Soup with Whole-Wheat Bread: A hearty and flavorful soup packed with protein and fiber.
- Salmon with Lemon Dill Sauce and Quinoa: This dish showcases the benefits of fatty fish with a light and flavorful sauce.

- Black Bean Burgers with Sweet Potato Fries:
  A satisfying vegetarian option loaded with
  protein and fiber.

- Spiced Chickpea and Vegetable Curry with
  Brown Rice: A flavorful and aromatic curry
  packed with plant-based protein and
  vegetables.

Additional Tips:

- **Cooking Methods:** Opt for healthy
  cooking methods like grilling, baking,
  roasting, or steaming to preserve nutrients
  and reduce unhealthy fats.

- **Seasoning:** Use herbs and spices to add
  flavor instead of relying on salt. To keep your
  meals interesting, experiment with diverse
  flavor characteristics.

- **Portion Control:** Be mindful of portion
  sizes to maintain a healthy calorie intake.

- **Enjoy the Journey:** Cooking and eating healthy meals should be an enjoyable experience. Take time to savor your food and appreciate the benefits it provides for your body.

By incorporating these recipes and tips into your routine, you can build a heart-healthy lifestyle that supports continued recovery and lifelong well-being

Recipes: Heart-Healthy Delights

This section features delicious and heart-healthy recipes that are perfect for incorporating into your continued recovery plan:

1. Mediterranean Chicken with Roasted Vegetables:

This dish is a symphony of flavors and textures, combining lean protein with colorful vegetables and the heart-healthy benefits of olive oil.

Ingredients:

- 2 boneless, skinless chicken breasts
- 1 tablespoon olive oil
- 1 teaspoon dried oregano
- ½ teaspoon garlic powder
- Salt and pepper to taste
- 1 bell pepper (red, yellow, or orange), sliced
- 1 medium zucchini, sliced
- 1 red onion, sliced
- 1 cup cherry tomatoes
- ¼ cup crumbled feta cheese (optional)
- Fresh parsley, chopped (for garnish)

Instructions:

1. Preheat the oven to 400°F (200°C).

2. In a bowl, toss chicken breasts with olive oil, oregano, garlic powder, salt, and pepper.

3. Place the chicken on a baking pan in a single layer.

4. Scatter the sliced vegetables (bell pepper, zucchini, onion, and cherry tomatoes) around the chicken.

5. Bake for 20-25 minutes, or until chicken is cooked through and vegetables are tender-crisp.

6. Sprinkle with crumbled feta cheese (if using) and fresh parsley before serving.

2. Vegetarian Chili with Whole-Wheat Bread:

This filling and healthful soup has a substantial, delicious base and is loaded with protein and fiber.

Ingredients:

- 1 tablespoon olive oil
- 1 onion, chopped
- 2 cloves garlic, minced
- 1 green bell pepper, chopped
- 1 (15 oz) can diced tomatoes, undrained
- 1 (15 oz) can kidney beans, rinsed and drained
- 1 (15 oz) can black beans, rinsed and drained
- 1 cup vegetable broth
- 1 teaspoon chili powder
- ½ teaspoon cumin
- ¼ teaspoon smoked paprika

- Salt and pepper to taste
- Chopped fresh cilantro (optional, for garnish)
- Whole-wheat bread slices

Instructions:

1. In a big pot, warm up the olive oil over medium heat.
2. Add the onion and simmer for about 5 minutes, or until softened.
3. Stir in garlic and bell pepper, cook for an additional minute.
4. Add diced tomatoes, kidney beans, black beans, vegetable broth, chili powder, cumin, smoked paprika, salt, and pepper.
5. Bring to a boil, then reduce heat and simmer for 15-20 minutes, or until flavors meld.
6. Serve hot in bowls with a side of whole-wheat bread for dipping.

7. Optionally garnish with chopped fresh cilantro.

3. Baked Fish with Lemon Dill Sauce and Quinoa:

This recipe showcases the heart-healthy benefits of fatty fish with a light and flavorful lemon dill sauce.

Ingredients:

- 2 salmon filets (4-6 ounces each)
- Salt and pepper to taste
- 1 tablespoon olive oil
- 1 tablespoon lemon juice
- ¼ cup chicken broth (low-sodium)
- 1 tablespoon chopped fresh dill
- 1 cup cooked quinoa

Instructions:

1. Preheat the oven to 400°F (200°C).

2. Season salmon filets with salt and pepper.

3. In a small bowl, whisk together olive oil, lemon juice, chicken broth, and fresh dill.

4. Place salmon filets in a baking dish and pour the lemon dill sauce over them.

5. Bake for 15-20 minutes, or until salmon is cooked through and flakes easily with a fork.

6. Serve over a bed of cooked quinoa for a complete meal.

Chapter 7: Brain-Boosting Meals for Cognitive Function

Following a stroke, nourishing your brain is just as important as nourishing your body. This chapter explores the concept of "brain food" and equips you with delicious recipes that can support cognitive function and overall brain health.

Fueling Your Cognitive Powerhouse:

The brain is a sophisticated organ that needs a constant flow of nourishment to perform at its best. Here's how your diet can influence cognitive function:

- **Essential Nutrients:** Certain vitamins, minerals, and antioxidants play a crucial role in brain health. These include vitamin B12, omega-3 fatty acids, and antioxidants found in fruits and vegetables.

- **Blood Flow:** A healthy diet can promote healthy blood flow throughout the body, including the brain. This ensures proper delivery of oxygen and nutrients to brain cells.

- **Inflammation:** Chronic inflammation can have negative effects on brain function.You can fight this by including anti-inflammatory items in your diet.

Brain-Boosting Food Choices:

- **Fatty Fish:** Fatty fish like salmon, tuna, and mackerel are rich in omega-3 fatty acids, which are essential for brain cell health and function.

- **Berries:** These colorful fruits are packed with antioxidants that protect brain cells from damage.

- **Leafy Green Vegetables:** Leafy greens like kale, spinach, and collard greens are loaded with vitamins and minerals that support cognitive function.

- **Nuts and Seeds:** Nuts and seeds are a great source of healthy fats, vitamin E, and other brain-boosting nutrients.

- **Whole Grains:** Whole grains provide sustained energy and a steady supply of glucose, the brain's preferred fuel source.

Sample Recipes: Brainpower Delights:

This section offers a variety of delicious and brain-boosting recipes to tantalize your taste buds and support cognitive health:

- **Salmon with Roasted Brussels Sprouts and Quinoa:** A one-pan meal featuring brain-healthy salmon and antioxidant-rich Brussels sprouts.

- **Berry Smoothie with Spinach and Nuts:** A refreshing and nutrient-packed smoothie packed with brain-boosting ingredients.

- **Lentil and Walnut Salad with Lemon Vinaigrette:** A hearty and satisfying salad that combines plant-based protein with healthy fats and fiber.

- **Chicken Stir-Fry with Broccoli and Brown Rice:** A quick and customizable stir-fry packed with brain-healthy vegetables and lean protein.

- **Whole-Wheat Pasta with Lentil Bolognese Sauce:** A flavorful vegetarian twist on a classic dish, providing protein, fiber, and essential nutrients.

Additional Tips:

- **Stay Hydrated:** Drinking plenty of water throughout the day is crucial for optimal brain function.

- **Mindful Eating:** Be aware of your body's signals of hunger and fullness. Eat slowly and savor your food to promote a healthy relationship with food.

- **Challenge Your Brain:** Engage in mentally stimulating activities like puzzles, games, or learning a new skill. This can help keep your brain sharp and improve cognitive function.

By incorporating these strategies, you can create a holistic approach to brain health and cognitive well-being after a stroke.

Recipes: Brainpower Delights

This section features delicious and brain-boosting recipes designed to tantalize your taste buds and support cognitive health:

1. Lentil and Walnut Salad with Lemon Vinaigrette:

This hearty and satisfying salad combines plant-based protein with healthy fats and fiber, making it a complete and brain-nourishing meal.

Ingredients:

- 1 cup cooked lentils (brown or green lentils work well)
- ½ cup chopped walnuts

- 1 cup baby spinach or mixed greens

- ½ cup cherry tomatoes, halved

- ¼ cup crumbled feta cheese (optional)

- ¼ cup chopped red onion

For the Lemon Vinaigrette:

- 2 tablespoons olive oil

- 1 tablespoon lemon juice

- 1 teaspoon Dijon mustard

- ½ teaspoon honey

- Salt and pepper to taste

Instructions:

1. In a large bowl, combine cooked lentils, walnuts, spinach, cherry tomatoes, and red onion.

2. To make the vinaigrette, whisk together olive oil, lemon juice, Dijon mustard, honey, salt, and pepper in a small bowl.

3. Drizzle the salad with the vinaigrette and
    toss to coat.

4. Top with crumbled feta cheese (if using) and
    serve.

2. Berry Oatmeal with Walnuts and Chia Seeds:

This recipe offers a delightful and brain-boosting breakfast option. Packed with antioxidants from berries, fiber from oatmeal, and healthy fats from walnuts and chia seeds, it fuels your brain for the day.

Ingredients:

- ½ cup rolled oats
- 1 cup milk (dairy or plant-based)

- ¼ cup mixed berries (fresh or frozen)

- 1 tablespoon chopped walnuts

- 1 tablespoon chia seeds

- Honey or maple syrup to taste (optional)

Instructions:

1. In a saucepan, combine rolled oats, milk, and a pinch of salt.

2. Bring to a boil over medium heat, then reduce heat and simmer for 5-7 minutes, or until oats are cooked through and creamy.

3. Remove from heat and stir in the mixed berries, walnuts, and chia seeds.

4. Drizzle with honey or maple syrup for additional sweetness (optional).

5. Serve warm and enjoy!

3. Salmon with Roasted Brussels Sprouts and Quinoa:

This one-pan meal features brain-healthy salmon and antioxidant-rich Brussels sprouts for a convenient and nutritious dinner.

Ingredients:

- 2 salmon filets (4-6 ounces each)
- 1 tablespoon olive oil
- Salt and pepper to taste
- 1 cup Brussels sprouts, trimmed and halved
- 1 cup cooked quinoa
- 1 lemon, sliced

Instructions:

1. Preheat the oven to 400°F (200°C).

2. In a baking dish, toss Brussels sprouts with olive oil, salt, and pepper.

3. Arrange salmon filets on top of the Brussels sprouts.

4. Place lemon slices around the salmon and dish.

5. Bake for 15-20 minutes, or until salmon is cooked through and flakes easily with a fork and Brussels sprouts are tender-crisp.

6. Serve immediately with the roasted Brussels sprouts and cooked quinoa.

Chapter 8: Easy and Adaptable Meals for Busy Lifestyles

Juggling work, family, and social commitments can leave little time for elaborate meal preparation. This chapter focuses on creating delicious and nutritious meals that are both easy to make and adaptable to your busy lifestyle.

Strategies for Success:

- **Planning is Key:** Dedicate some time each week to plan your meals and create a grocery list.You'll be able to steer clear of bad last-minute choices by doing this.

- **Batch Cooking:** Cook larger portions of certain dishes on the weekend and portion them out for easy reheating throughout the week.

- **Smart Leftovers:** Leftovers can be your friend! Repurpose them into new and exciting meals the next day.

- **Embrace Simplicity:** Don't be afraid of simple meals. A well-balanced salad with a lean protein source can be a healthy and satisfying lunch option.

- **Utilize Shortcuts:** Utilize pre-cut vegetables, frozen fruits, or canned beans to save time without sacrificing nutrition.

Easy and Adaptable Recipes:

This section offers a variety of recipes that are quick to prepare and can be easily customized to your preferences and dietary needs:

- **Sheet Pan Dinners:** Toss your favorite protein and vegetables together on a sheet pan, drizzle with olive oil and seasonings, and bake for a hassle-free one-pan meal.

- **Stir-Fry Magic:** Stir-fries are a perfect canvas for customization. Choose your favorite protein, vegetables, and sauce for a quick and flavorful meal.

- **Big Batch Soups and Stews:** Prepare a large pot of soup or stew on the weekend. It will provide you with healthy lunches or dinners throughout the week and freezes well for future use.

- **Power Bowls:** Power bowls offer endless possibilities. Start with a base of quinoa, brown rice, or leafy greens, then add your favorite protein, vegetables, and toppings for a complete and satisfying meal.

- **Breakfast for Dinner:** Sometimes, breakfast for dinner is just what the busy schedule calls for. Opt for a healthy omelet, whole-wheat pancakes with fruit, or yogurt parfaits for a quick and satisfying meal.

Additional Tips:

- **Prep Work Matters:** Spend 15-20 minutes on a weekend chopping vegetables, cooking a pot of brown rice, or prepping some lean protein for the week. When you're pressed for time during the week, this will save you time.

- **Get Creative with Leftovers:** Leftover chicken can be transformed into a delicious chicken salad sandwich or chicken stir-fry. Leftover roasted vegetables can be added to omelets or salads.

- **Cook Once, Eat Twice:** When preparing a recipe, consider doubling the batch and freezing half for another night. This minimizes cooking time in the long run.

- **Involve the Family: Get** your family involved in meal planning and preparation. This can be a fun bonding experience and encourages healthy eating habits for everyone.

By incorporating these strategies and recipes, you can conquer your busy schedule without compromising on your well-being. Enjoy the journey of creating delicious and nutritious meals that fit perfectly into your life!

Recipes: Easy Wins for Busy Lives

This section features a variety of quick and adaptable recipes that are perfect for busy schedules. These "Easy Wins" are designed to be delicious, nutritious, and require minimal prep or cleanup time.

1. Sheet Pan Fajitas: (One-Pot Wonder)

This vibrant and flavorful dish comes together on a single sheet pan, minimizing cleanup.

Ingredients:

- 1 pound boneless, skinless chicken breasts or thighs, sliced
- 1 bell pepper (red, yellow, or orange), sliced
- 1 onion, sliced
- 1 tablespoon olive oil
- 1 teaspoon chili powder

- ½ teaspoon cumin

- ¼ teaspoon smoked paprika

- Salt and pepper to taste

- Optional Toppings: Warmed tortillas, shredded cheese, salsa, guacamole, sour cream

Instructions:

1. Preheat the oven to 400°F (200°C).
2. In a large bowl, toss chicken pieces, bell pepper slices, and onion slices with olive oil, chili powder, cumin, smoked paprika, salt, and pepper.
3. Spread the seasoned ingredients on a rimmed baking sheet.
4. Bake for 20-25 minutes, or until chicken is cooked through and vegetables are tender-crisp.
5. Serve hot with your favorite fajita toppings.

Leftover Makeover: Leftover fajita chicken can be repurposed into a delicious chicken quesadilla or burrito bowl the next day.

2. Leftover Salmon Scramble: (Leftover Makeover)

This recipe transforms leftover salmon into a protein-packed and flavorful breakfast scramble.

Ingredients:

- 1 cup cooked and flaked salmon
- 2 eggs, beaten
- ½ cup chopped vegetables (such as bell pepper, onion, or spinach)
- 1 tablespoon chopped fresh herbs (such as dill or chives)
- Salt and pepper to taste
- Optional Toppings: Chopped avocado, crumbled feta cheese, whole-wheat toast

Instructions:

1. In a non-stick pan, heat a pat of butter or drizzle of olive oil over medium heat.

2. Add the chopped vegetables and cook until softened, about 3 minutes.

3. Add the flaked salmon and stir to combine.

4. Pour in the beaten eggs and cook, stirring occasionally, until the eggs are set and cooked through.

5. Season with salt and pepper to taste.

6. Serve immediately with your favorite toppings.

3. Overnight Oats with Berries and Nuts: (Quick Breakfast Idea)

This simple recipe requires minimal prep and can be enjoyed throughout the week.

Ingredients:

- ½ cup rolled oats
- 1 cup milk (dairy or plant-based)
- ¼ cup plain yogurt
- ¼ cup mixed berries (fresh or frozen)
- 1 tablespoon chopped nuts (such as almonds or walnuts)
- Honey or maple syrup to taste (optional)

Instructions:

1. In a mason jar or container, combine rolled oats, milk, yogurt, berries, and chopped nuts.

2. Stir well, cover, and refrigerate overnight.

3. In the morning, stir again and enjoy the cold. Drizzle with honey or maple syrup for additional sweetness (optional).

Chapter 9: Delicious Desserts You Can Enjoy on a Stroke Diet

Following a stroke, indulging in your sweet tooth doesn't have to be off-limits. This chapter explores delicious and healthy dessert options that are perfectly suitable for a stroke diet. These recipes focus on:

- **Natural Sweeteners:** Limiting added sugar while still enjoying sweetness with natural options like fruits, dates, and honey.
- **Healthy Fats:** Incorporating healthy fats like nuts, seeds, and avocado for satiety and additional nutrients.

- **Portion Control:** Enjoying desserts in moderation to maintain a balanced diet.

Sweet Treats Done Right:

Here are some general tips for creating healthy and satisfying desserts on a stroke diet:

- **Focus on Fruits:** Fruits are a natural source of sweetness and packed with vitamins, minerals, and fiber. Enjoy them fresh, frozen, or baked into delicious desserts.
- **Get Creative with Spices:** Spices like cinnamon, nutmeg, and ginger can add depth of flavor and reduce your reliance on added sugar.

- **Experiment with Healthy Fats:** Healthy fats like avocado, nut butters, and chia seeds can add creaminess and richness to desserts without compromising taste or nutrition.

- **Control Portions:** Enjoy your favorite desserts, but be mindful of portion sizes. A small serving can satisfy your sweet tooth without going overboard.

Sample Dessert Delights:

This section offers a variety of delicious and healthy dessert options to satisfy your cravings:

- **Baked Apples with Cinnamon and Walnuts:** A classic and comforting dessert featuring naturally sweet apples with a hint of cinnamon and a satisfying crunch from walnuts.

- **Frozen Yogurt Parfaits with Berries and Granola:** A refreshing and layered dessert with protein-rich yogurt, antioxidant-rich berries, and a touch of granola for added texture.

- **Chocolate Avocado Mousse:** This decadent and healthy mousse gets its creaminess from avocado and a touch of natural sweetness from dates or honey. A sprinkle of cocoa powder adds a satisfying chocolatey flavor.

- **Chia Seed Pudding with Mango and Coconut Milk:** This pudding is packed with fiber and healthy fats for a satisfying dessert. The natural sweetness of mango and the creaminess of coconut milk create a delightful combination.

- **Poached Pears with a Spiced Honey Glaze:** This elegant dessert features poached pears drizzled with a flavorful honey glaze infused with warming spices like cinnamon and cloves.

Additional Tips:

- **Planning is Key:** Plan your desserts in advance to avoid unhealthy temptations. Having healthy options readily available can help you make smart choices.

- **Get the Family Involved**: Involve your family in creating healthy dessert options. For those involved, this may be an enjoyable and instructive experience.

- **Celebrate Special Occasions:** Special occasions still deserve a sweet treat! Choose a healthy dessert recipe and enjoy it in moderation.

By incorporating these tips and recipes, you can satisfy your sweet tooth while maintaining a healthy lifestyle after a stroke.

Sample Dessert Delights: Sweet Treats for a Healthy You

This section features a variety of delicious and healthy dessert options that are perfect for satisfying your sweet tooth while following a stroke diet:

1. Simple Fruit Crumble:

A comforting classic with a healthy twist! This crumble features naturally sweet seasonal fruits topped with a crunchy oat and nut crumble.

Ingredients:

- **For the Fruit Filling:**
  - 4 cups mixed fruits (such as apples, pears, berries)
  - 2 tablespoons cornstarch
  - 1/4 cup water
  - 1/4 cup honey or maple syrup
  - 1 teaspoon lemon juice
  - 1/2 teaspoon ground cinnamon
- **For the Oat Crumble:**
  - 1 cup rolled oats
  - 1/2 cup chopped nuts (such as almonds or walnuts)
  - 1/4 cup brown sugar (packed)
  - 3 tablespoons melted butter

Instructions:

1. Preheat the oven to 375°F (190°C).

2. In a bowl, combine the mixed fruits, cornstarch, water, honey, lemon juice, and cinnamon. Toss to coat.

3. Transfer the fruit mixture to a baking dish.

4. In a separate bowl, combine rolled oats, chopped nuts, brown sugar, and melted butter. Mix until crumbly.

5. Sprinkle the oat crumble topping evenly over the fruit filling.

6. Bake for 30-35 minutes, or until the fruit is bubbly and the crumble topping is golden brown.

7. Serve warm or at room temperature with a dollop of low-fat yogurt (optional).

2. Baked Apples with Cinnamon and Walnuts:

This timeless delight offers the taste of comfort food with a healthy twist. Baked apples are naturally sweet and filled with warming cinnamon, all topped with a satisfying crunch of walnuts.

Ingredients:

- 4 apples (such as Granny Smith, Honeycrisp)
- 1/4 cup chopped walnuts
- 2 tablespoons rolled oats
- 1 tablespoon honey or maple syrup
- 1 teaspoon ground cinnamon
- 1/4 teaspoon nutmeg (optional)

Instructions:

1. Preheat the oven to 375°F (190°C).

2. Core the apples, leaving a small bottom intact.

3. In a small bowl, combine chopped walnuts, rolled oats, honey, cinnamon, and nutmeg (if using).

4. Stuff the apple cores with the oat mixture.

5. Place the apples in a baking dish and add a splash of water to the bottom of the dish to prevent burning.

6. Bake for thirty to thirty-five minutes, until the apples are soft and the topping is browned.

7. Serve warm or at room temperature with a sprinkle of additional cinnamon (optional).

3. Creamy Yogurt Popsicles with Berries:

These cool and nutritious popsicles are ideal on a steamy summer's day. They offer a satisfying combination of creamy yogurt and antioxidant-rich berries.

Ingredients:

- 2 cups plain yogurt (Greek yogurt works well)
- 1/2 cup mixed berries (fresh or frozen)
- 1/4 cup honey or maple syrup (optional)

Instructions:

1. In a blender, combine yogurt, berries, and honey (if using). Blend until smooth.
2. Pour the mixture into popsicle molds.

3. Freeze for at least 4-6 hours, or until solid.

4. Enjoy these healthy and refreshing popsicles on a hot day!

Part 3: Essential Resources

This section equips you with valuable tools and resources to support your lifelong wellness journey after a stroke recovery.

Appendix: Helpful Charts and Cooking Tips

The appendix provides a collection of helpful charts and cooking tips to make healthy cooking a breeze:

Charts:

- **Food Exchange Chart:** This chart helps you understand portion sizes and create balanced meals by categorizing foods into different groups (carbohydrates, proteins, fats, etc.).

- **Seasoning Substitution Chart**: This chart provides substitutions for common seasonings, allowing you to experiment and adjust recipes to your taste preferences.

- **Salt Reduction Tips Chart:** This chart offers tips and substitutes for reducing sodium intake while maintaining flavor in your meals.

- **Healthy Cooking Methods Chart:** This chart showcases various healthy cooking methods (grilling, baking, steaming) along with their benefits and suitable foods.

Cooking Tips:

- **Meal Planning Hacks:** Learn time-saving strategies for meal planning, including creating a grocery list and prepping ingredients in advance.

- **Leftover Magic:** Discover creative ways to transform leftovers into new and exciting dishes, reducing food waste and saving time.

- **Flavor Boosting Techniques:** Explore tips and tricks for adding flavor to your meals without relying on excessive salt or unhealthy fats.

- **Kitchen Safety Essentials:** Review basic kitchen safety practices to ensure a safe and enjoyable cooking experience.

Additional Resources:

- **Consider exploring these organizations for further guidance:**
  - American Heart Association
  - American Stroke Association
  - Academy of Nutrition and Dietetics
  - National Institute on Deafness and Other Communication Disorders (For resources on swallowing difficulties)

Glossary of Stroke Diet Terms

Following a stroke, you may encounter new terms related to dietary recommendations. This glossary clarifies those terms to empower you to make informed choices:

- **Balanced Diet:** A diet that includes a variety of foods from all food groups (fruits, vegetables, whole grains, lean protein, healthy fats) in appropriate proportions.

- **Cholesterol**: A waxy substance found in the blood. High levels of LDL ("bad") cholesterol can contribute to plaque buildup in arteries, increasing the risk of stroke.

- **Fiber:** A type of carbohydrate found in plant-based foods that aids digestion and promotes feelings of fullness.

- **Healthy Fats:** Unsaturated fats, such as those found in olive oil, avocados, and nuts, can help lower bad cholesterol and improve heart health.

- **Portion Control:** Practicing mindful eating and consuming appropriate serving sizes to maintain a healthy weight and blood pressure.

- **Salt (Sodium):** Excessive sodium intake can raise blood pressure, a risk factor for stroke.

- **Saturated Fats:** Fats found in animal products and some processed foods. Limiting saturated fat intake can improve heart health.

- **Stroke Diet:** A general term for a dietary pattern that emphasizes healthy eating to promote recovery and reduce the risk of future strokes. It focuses on fruits, vegetables, whole grains, lean protein, and healthy fats while limiting saturated fat, sodium, and added sugar.

- **Sugar:** Excessive added sugar intake can contribute to weight gain and other health problems. Natural sugars found in fruits are generally less concerning.

Additional Terms:

- **Dysphagia:** Difficulty swallowing. A speech-language pathologist can provide guidance on safe swallowing techniques for individuals with dysphagia.
- **Food Exchange Chart:** A tool that categorizes foods into groups based on their nutrient content, helping with portion control and meal planning.

This glossary provides a starting point. If you have any questions or concerns about your specific dietary needs after a stroke, consult a registered dietitian or your healthcare provider.

Additional Resources for Stroke Recovery and Healthy Living

Beyond the information provided in this book, here are valuable resources to support your stroke recovery and overall well-being:

Government Organizations:

- **National Institute of Neurological Disorders and Stroke (NINDS):** Provides comprehensive information on stroke, including causes, symptoms, diagnosis, treatment, and rehabilitation.

- **Centers for Disease Control and Prevention (CDC):** Offers resources on stroke prevention, risk factors, and healthy lifestyle choices.

- **Office of Disease Prevention and Health Promotion (ODPHP):** Provides resources on healthy eating, physical activity, and chronic disease management, all of which are important for stroke recovery and prevention.

Stroke Associations:

- **American Stroke Association:** The leading voluntary health organization dedicated to fighting stroke. Offers information on stroke prevention, warning signs, treatment options, and support resources.

- **National Stroke Association:** Another patient-centered organization providing stroke information, support groups, and educational resources.

Non-Profit Organizations:

- **The American Heart Association:** Focuses on heart health, which is closely linked to stroke risk. Provides information on healthy living, risk factors, and stroke prevention strategies.

- **The Brain Trauma Foundation**: Offers resources on brain injury, including stroke, with a focus on research, education, and advocacy.

- **The Christopher & Dana Reeve Foundation:** Provides information and support for people living with paralysis, including those with stroke-related disabilities.

Online Support Groups:

- **Stroke Support Groups** - Stroke Association: Connects you with online communities of stroke survivors and caregivers for peer support and information sharing.

- **National Stroke Association Online Community:** Another online forum for stroke survivors and caregivers to connect, share experiences, and offer encouragement.

www.ingramcontent.com/pod-product-compliance
Lightning Source LLC
Chambersburg PA
CBHW071039250726
48653CB00005B/1899